THE PICTURE BOOK OF
CHRISTMAS

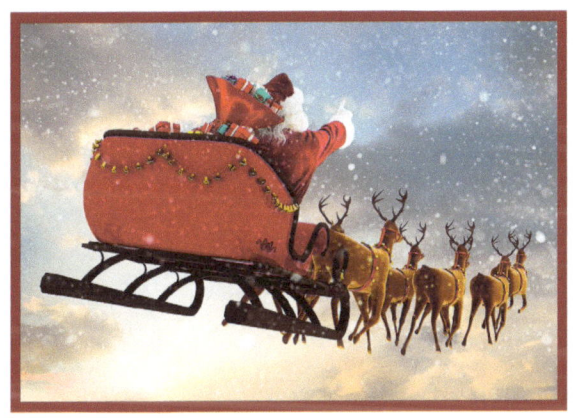

SUNNY STREET
BOOKS

Christmas Tree

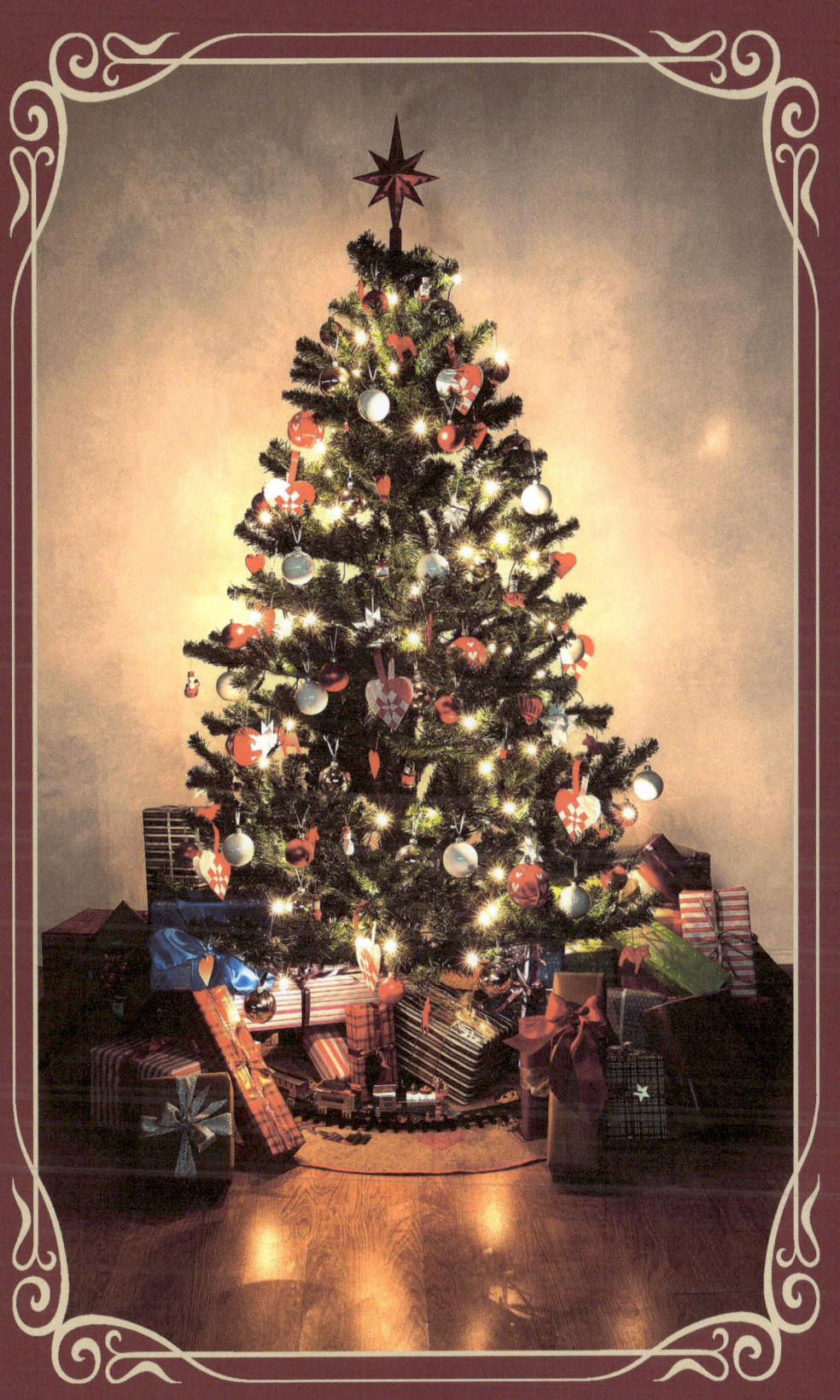

Christmas Cookies

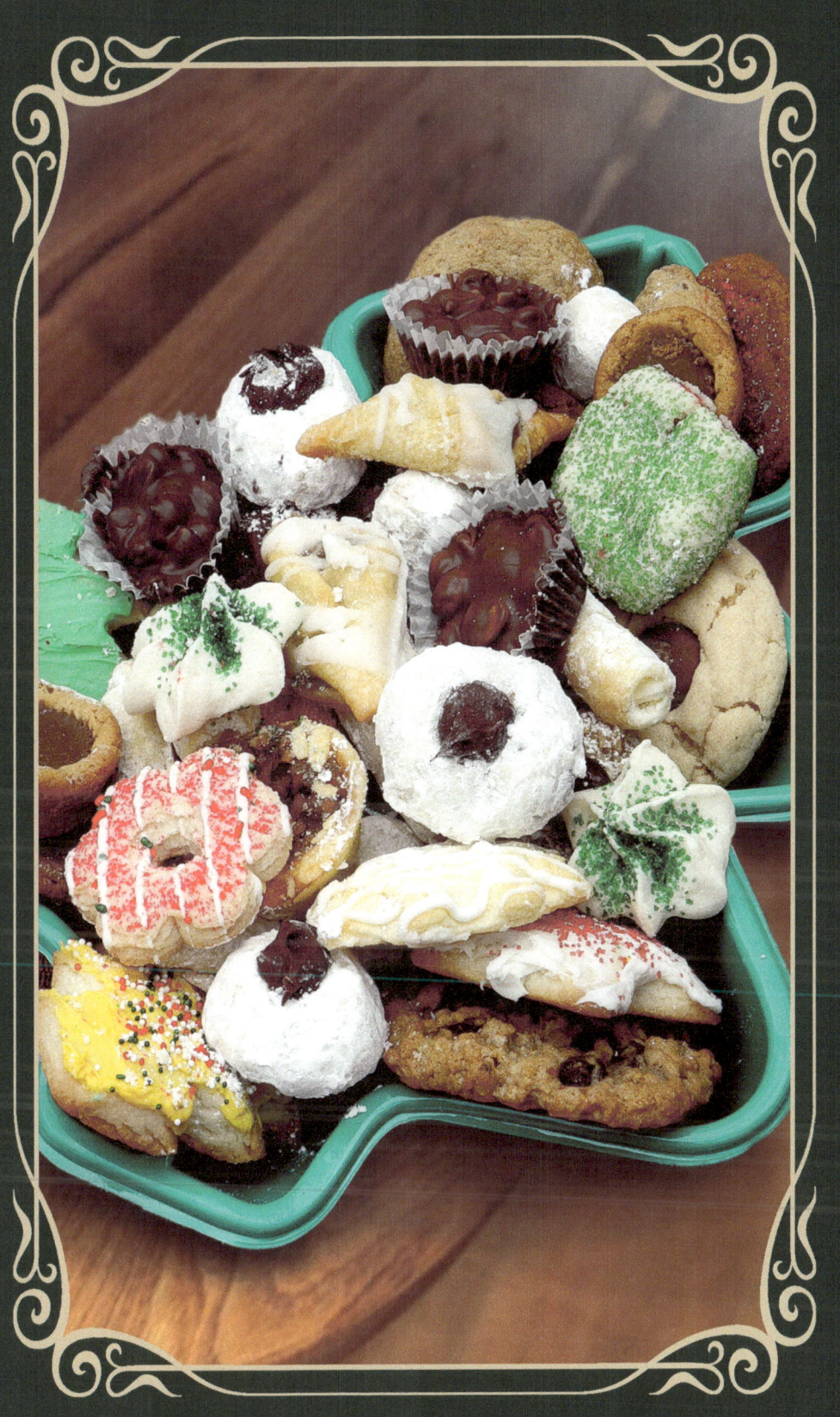

CANDY
CANES

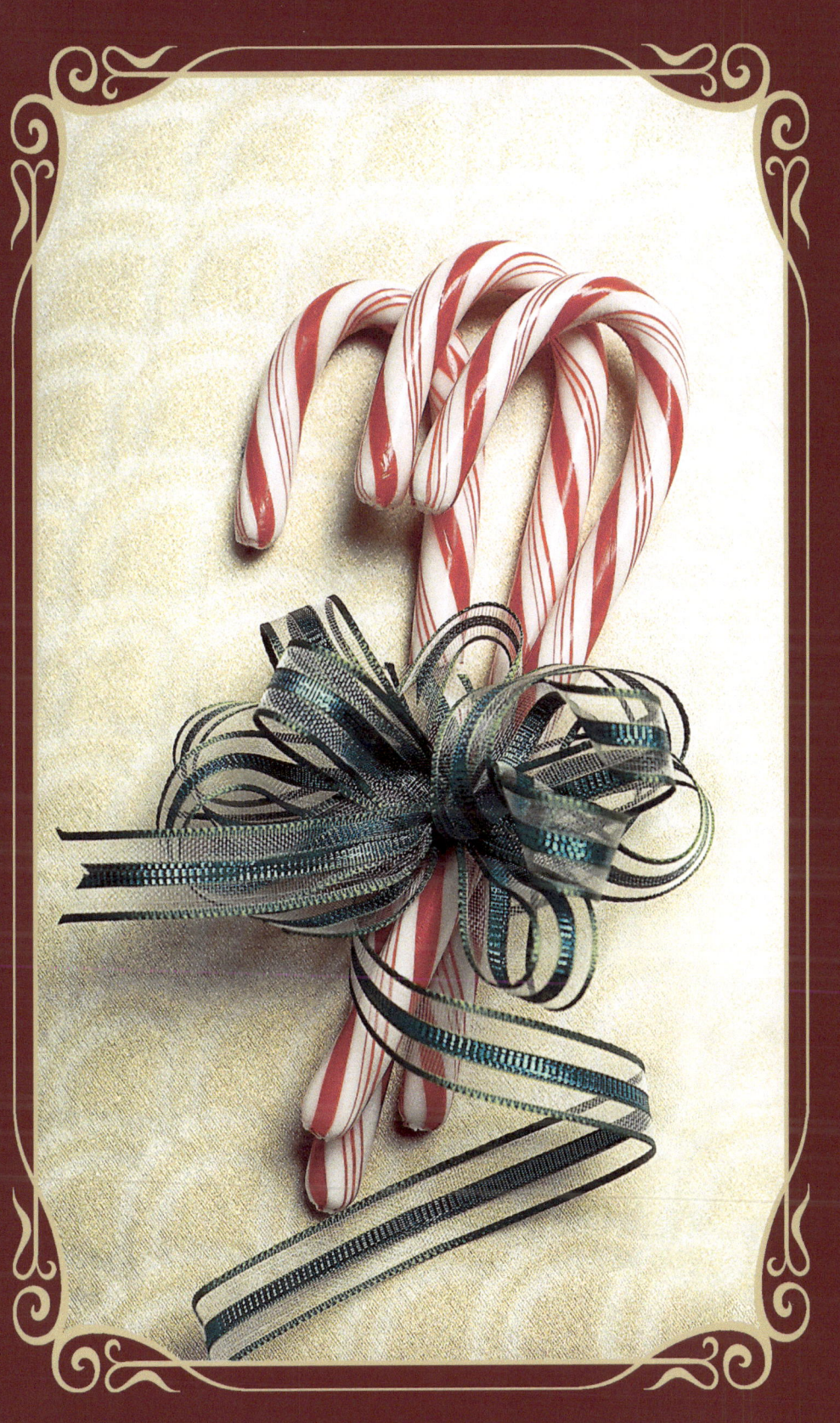

CHRISTMAS ANGEL

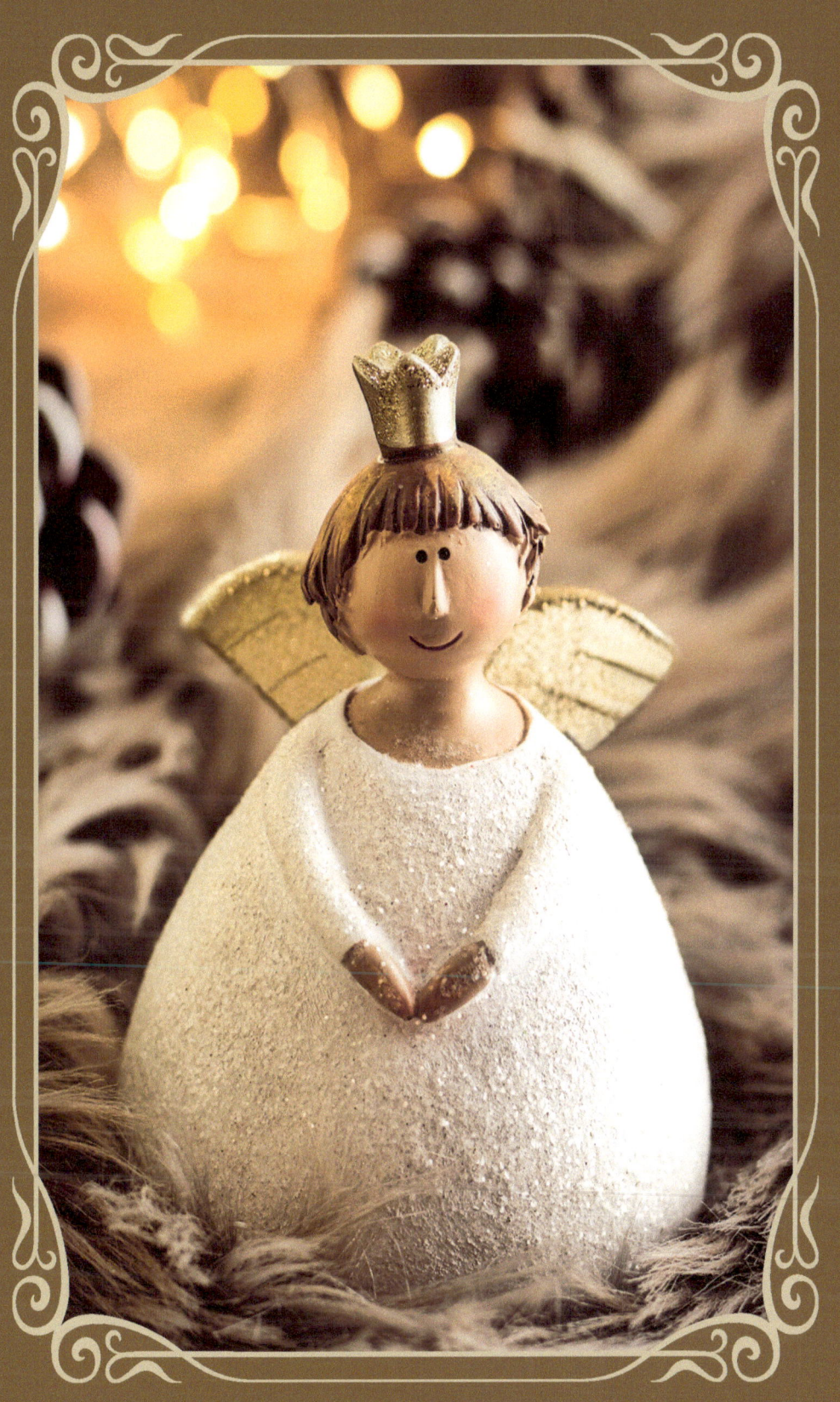

Santa Claus

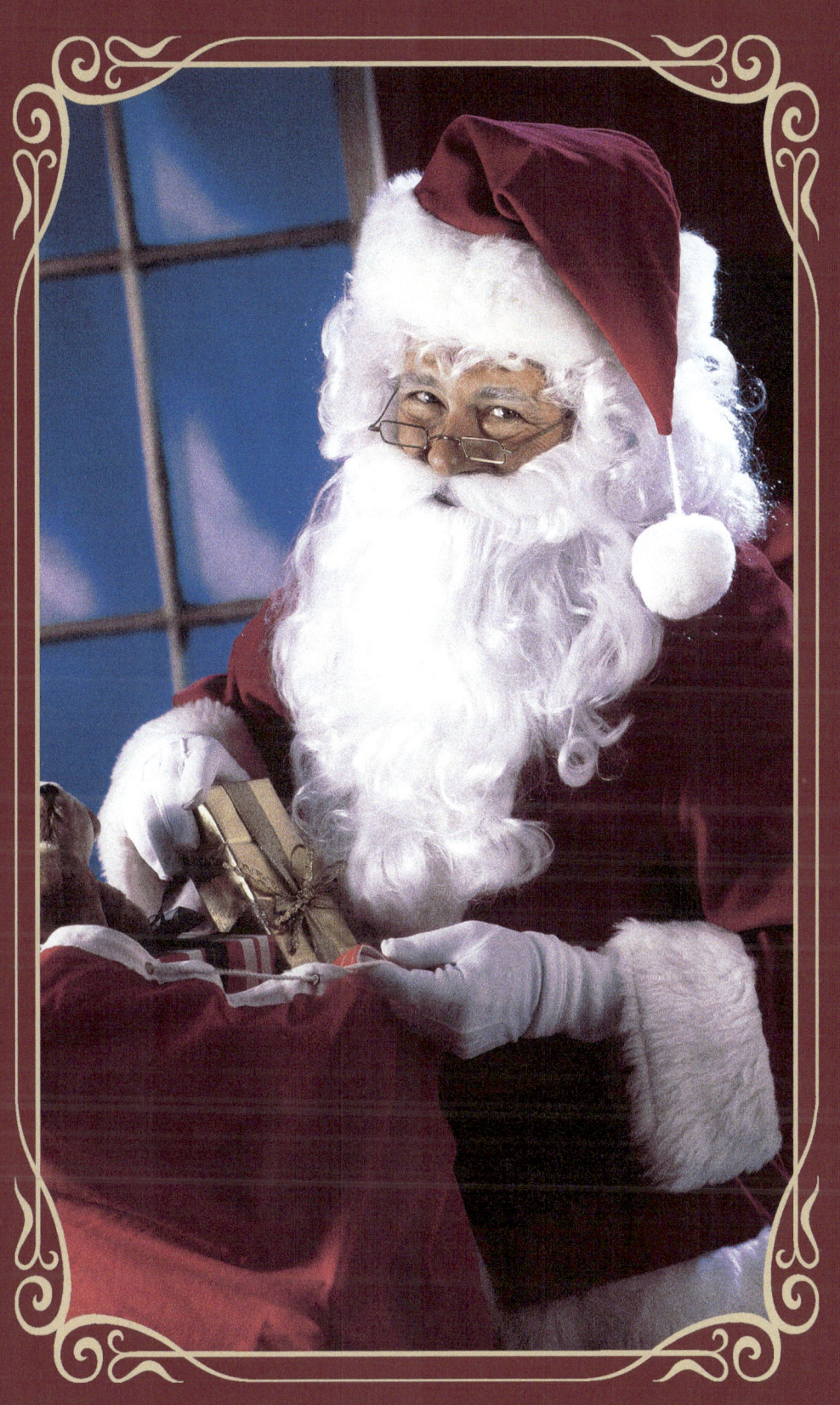

CHRISTMAS LIGHTS

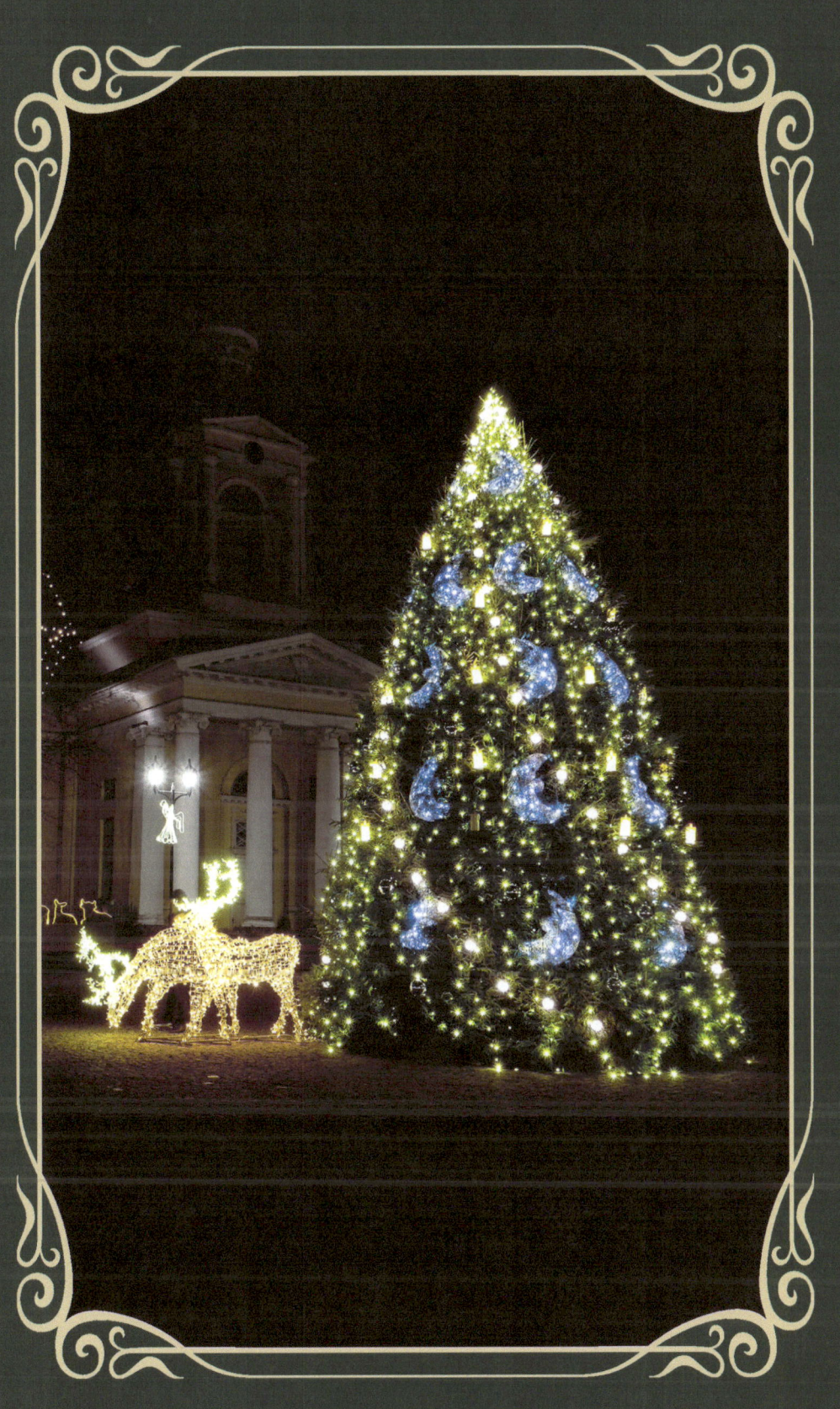

Reindeer

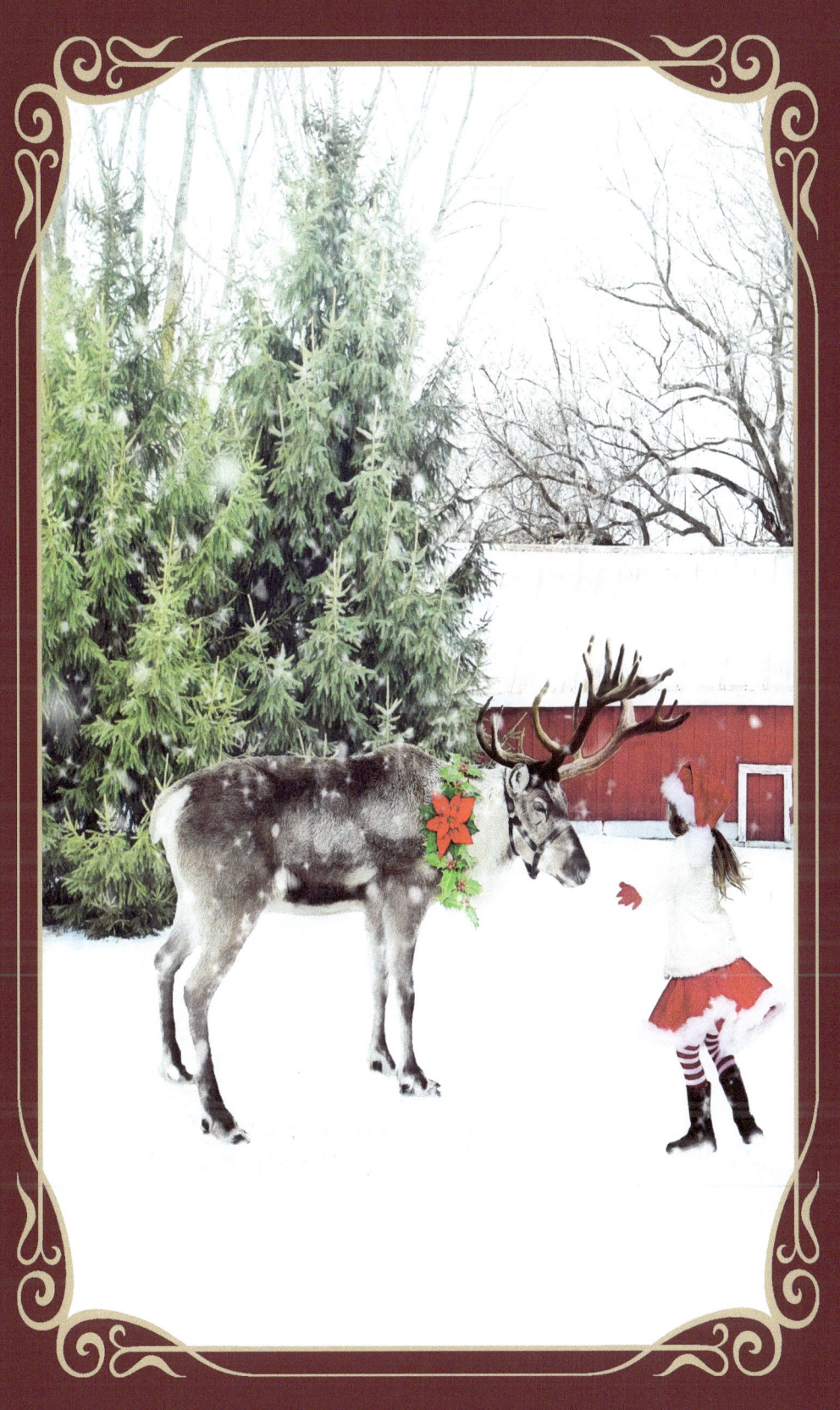

Sledding

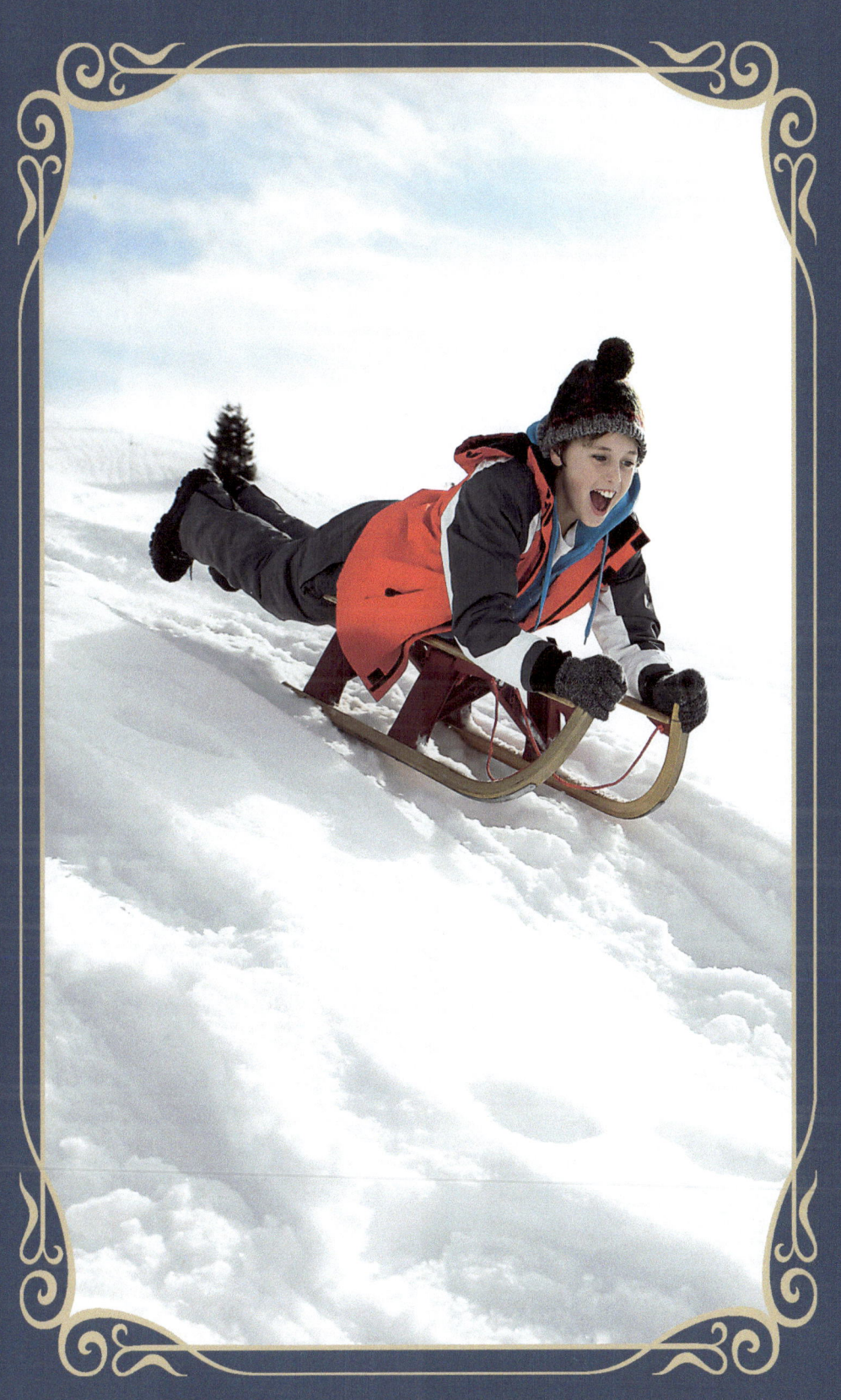

SNOWMAN

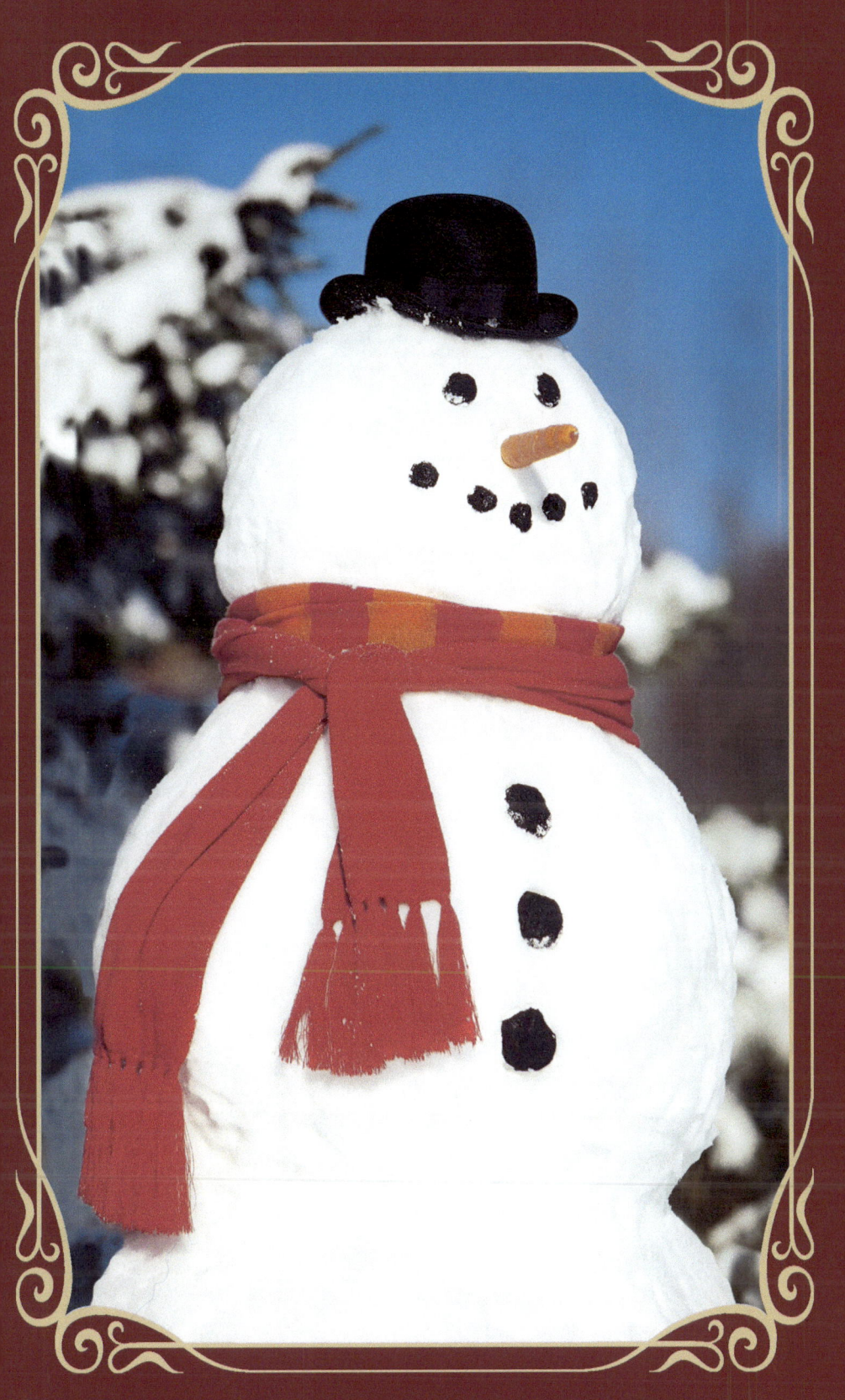

CHRISTMAS ORNAMENTS

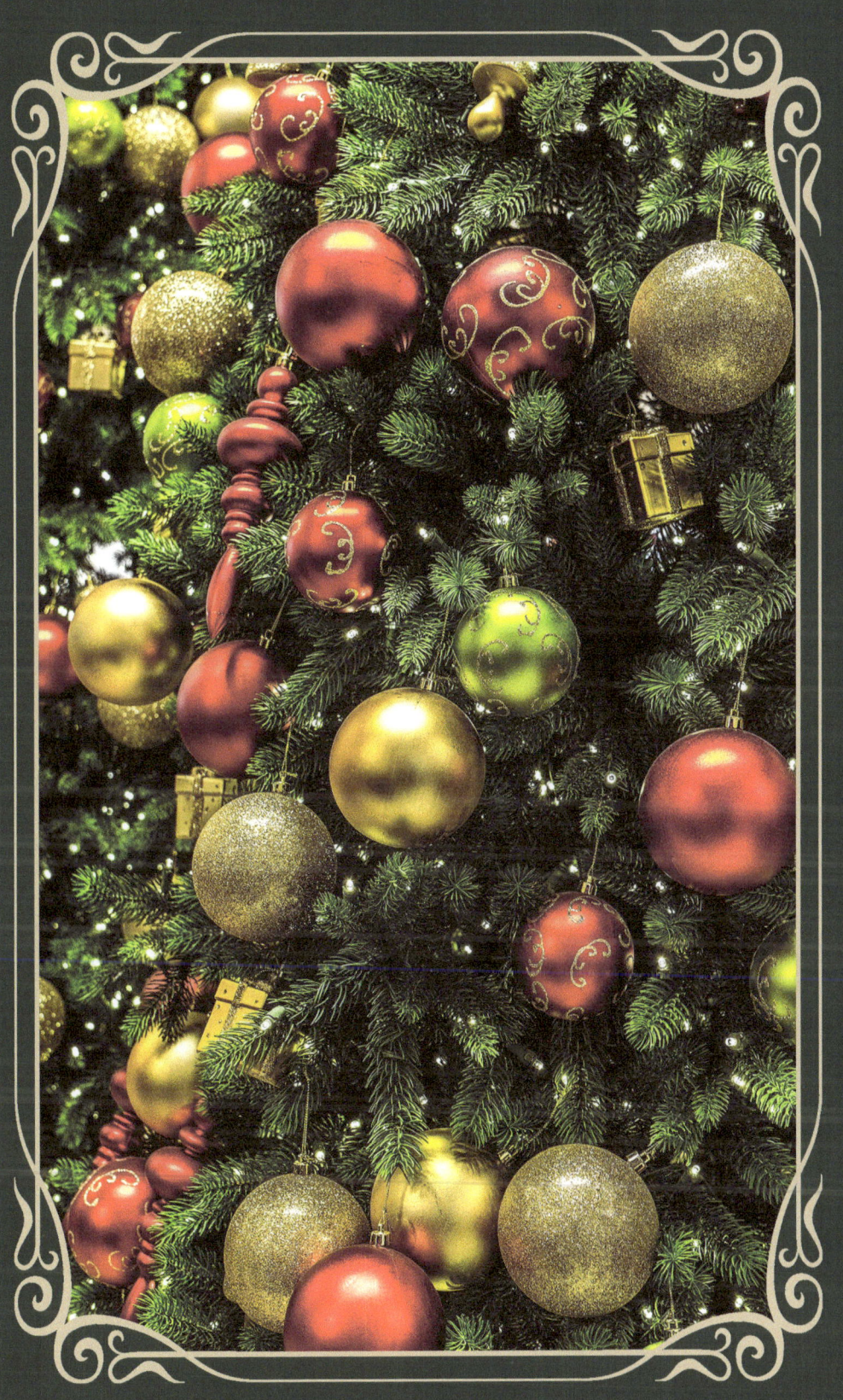

CHRISTMAS CANDLES

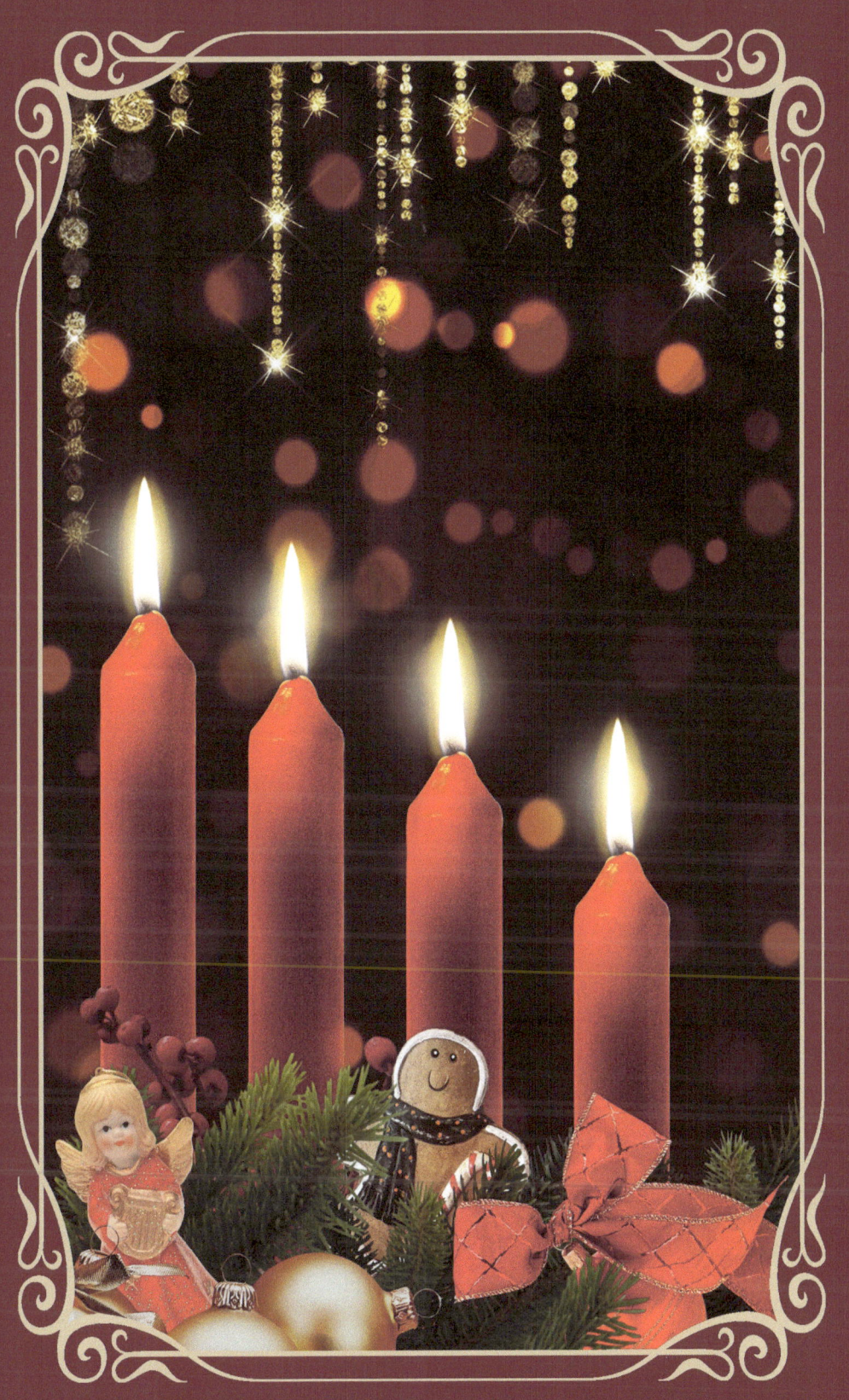

Gingerbread House

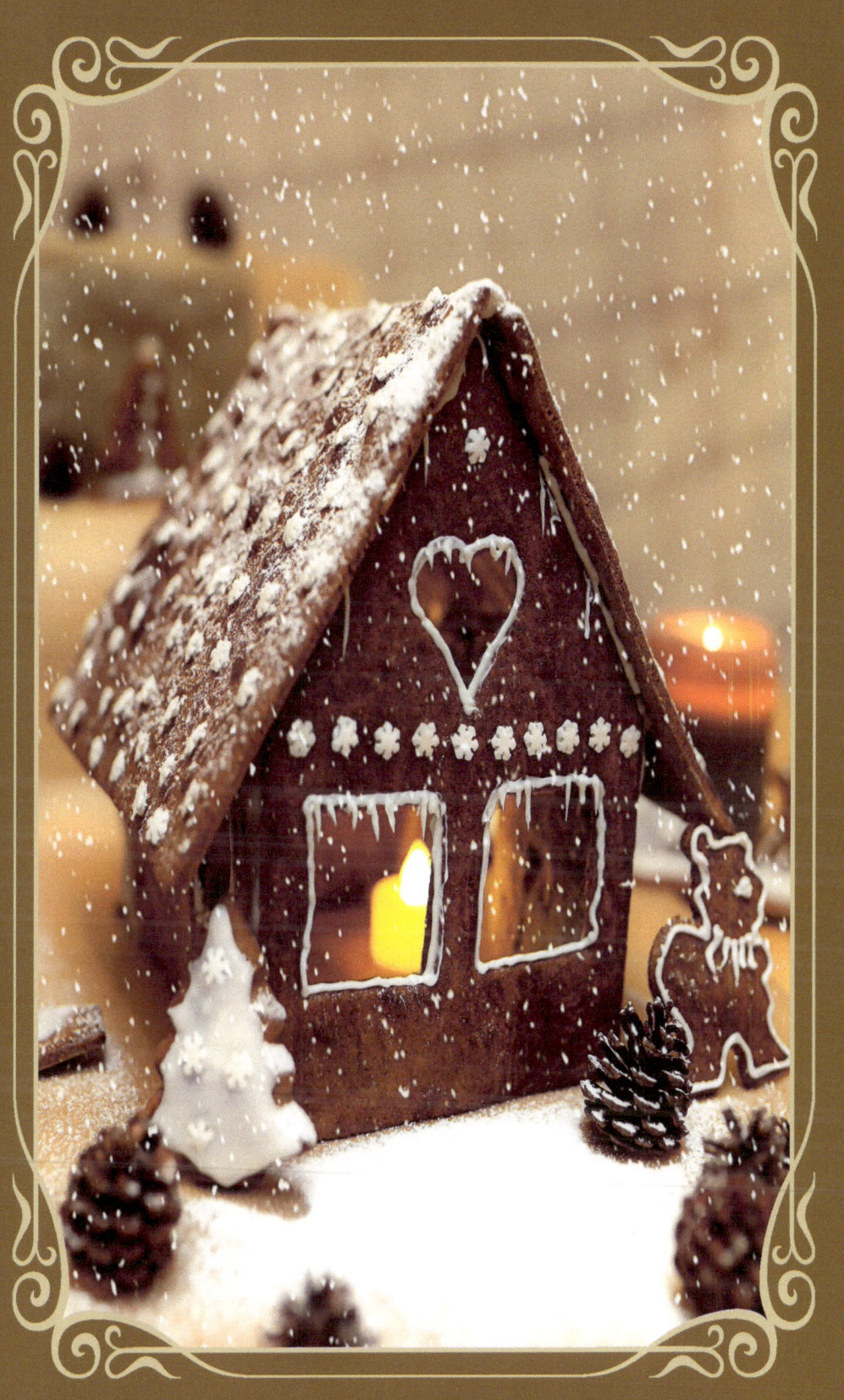

Christmas Stocking

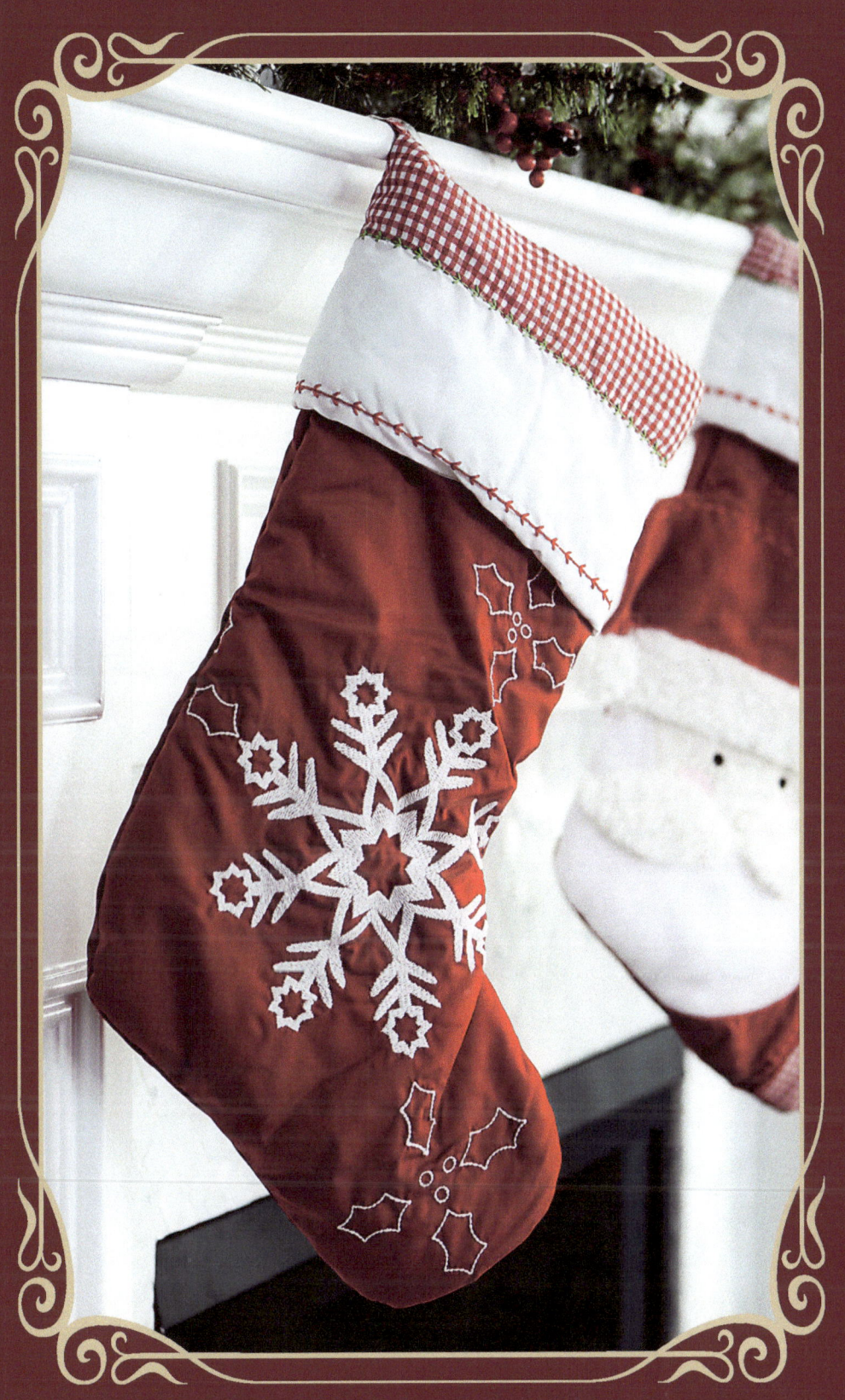

HOT
COCOA

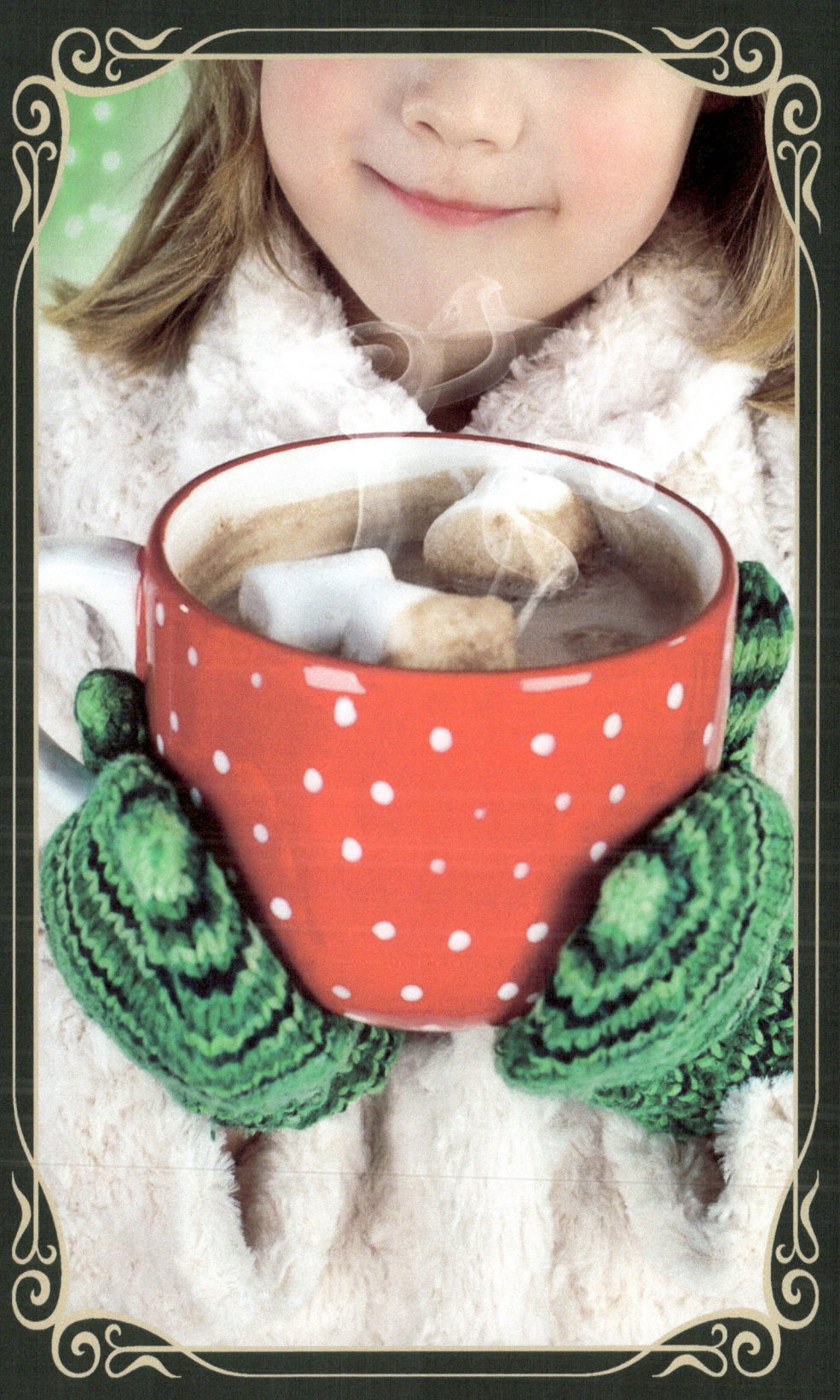

Christmas Dinner

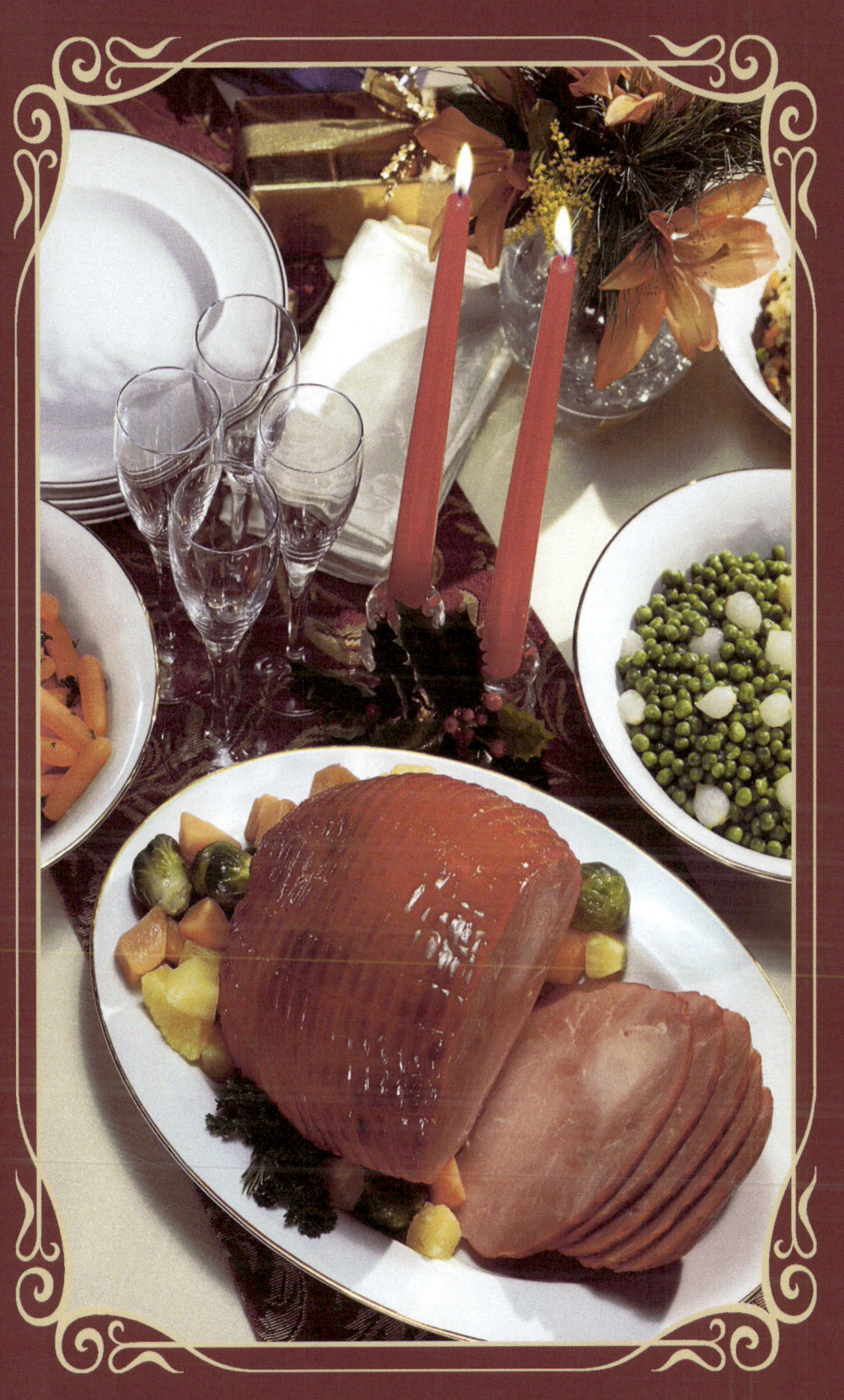

Snow

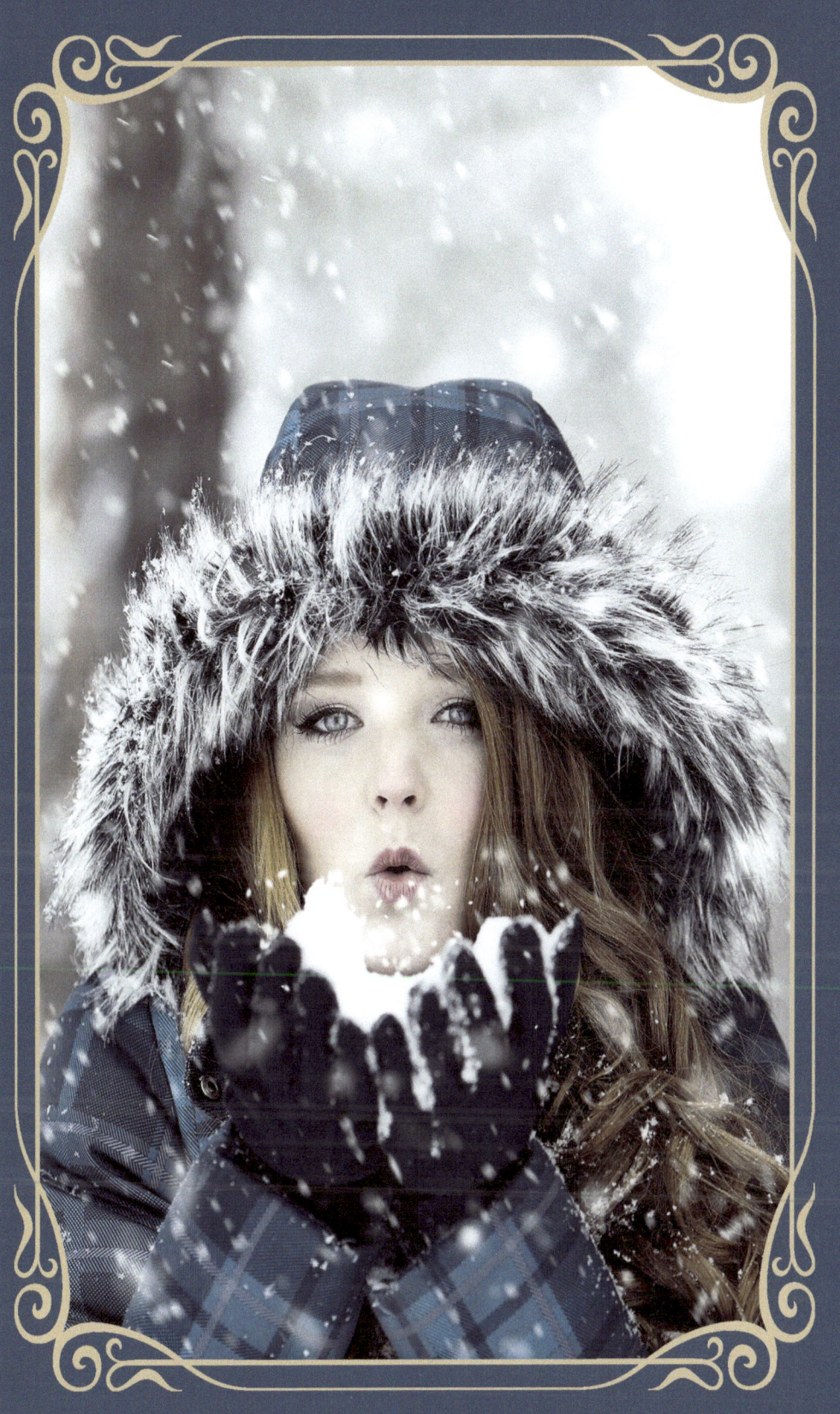

SANTA'S
SLEIGH

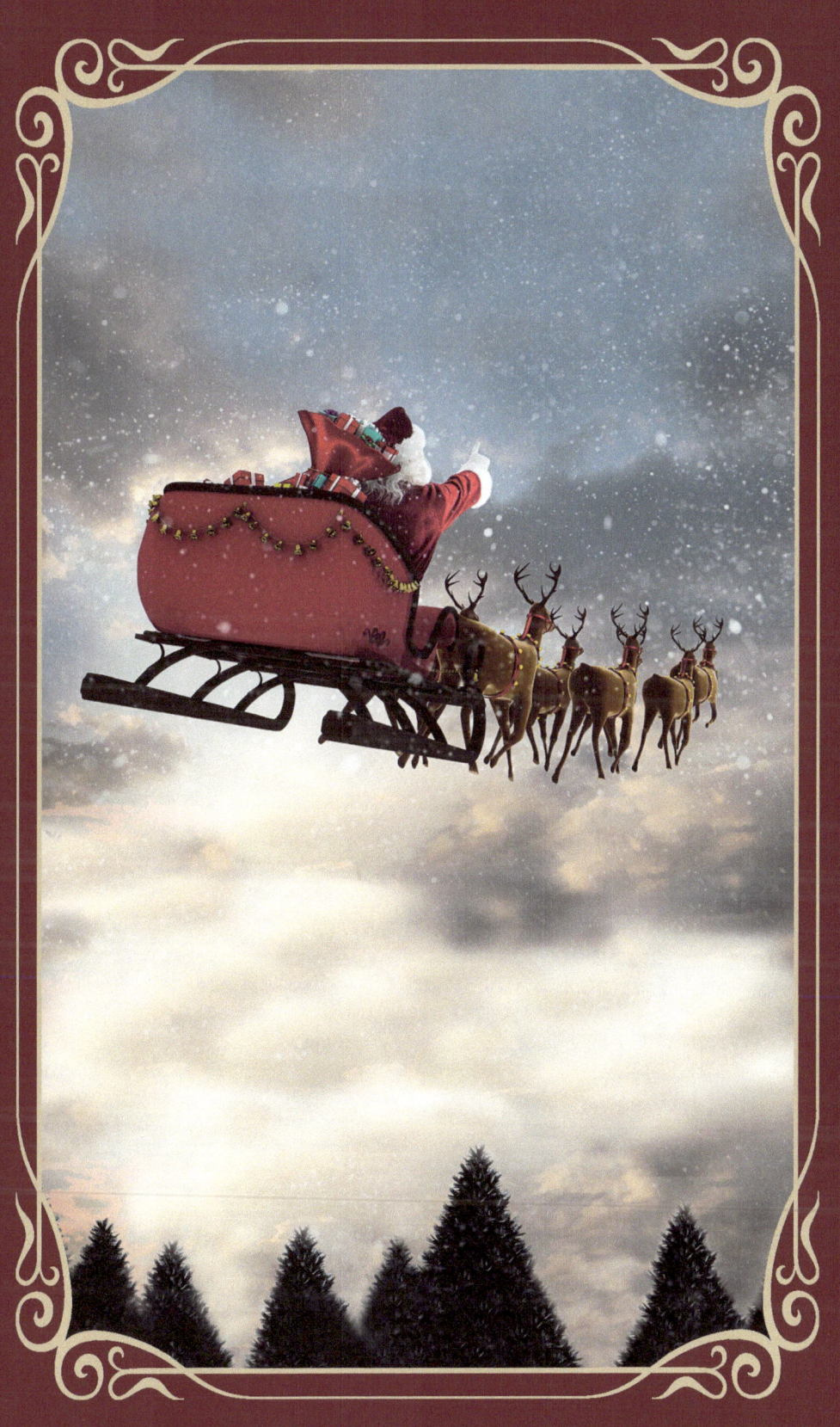

POINSETTAS

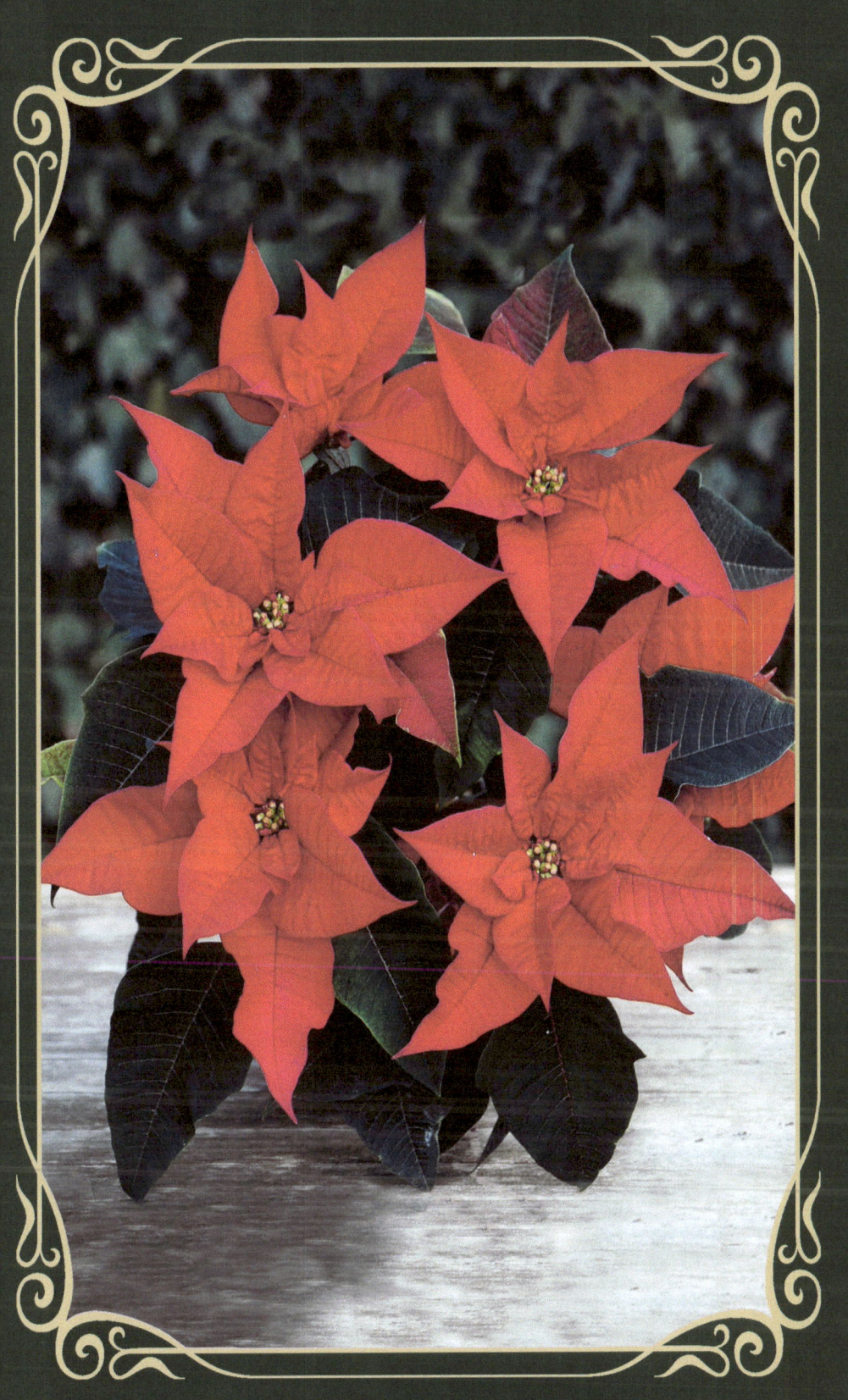

Nativity Scene

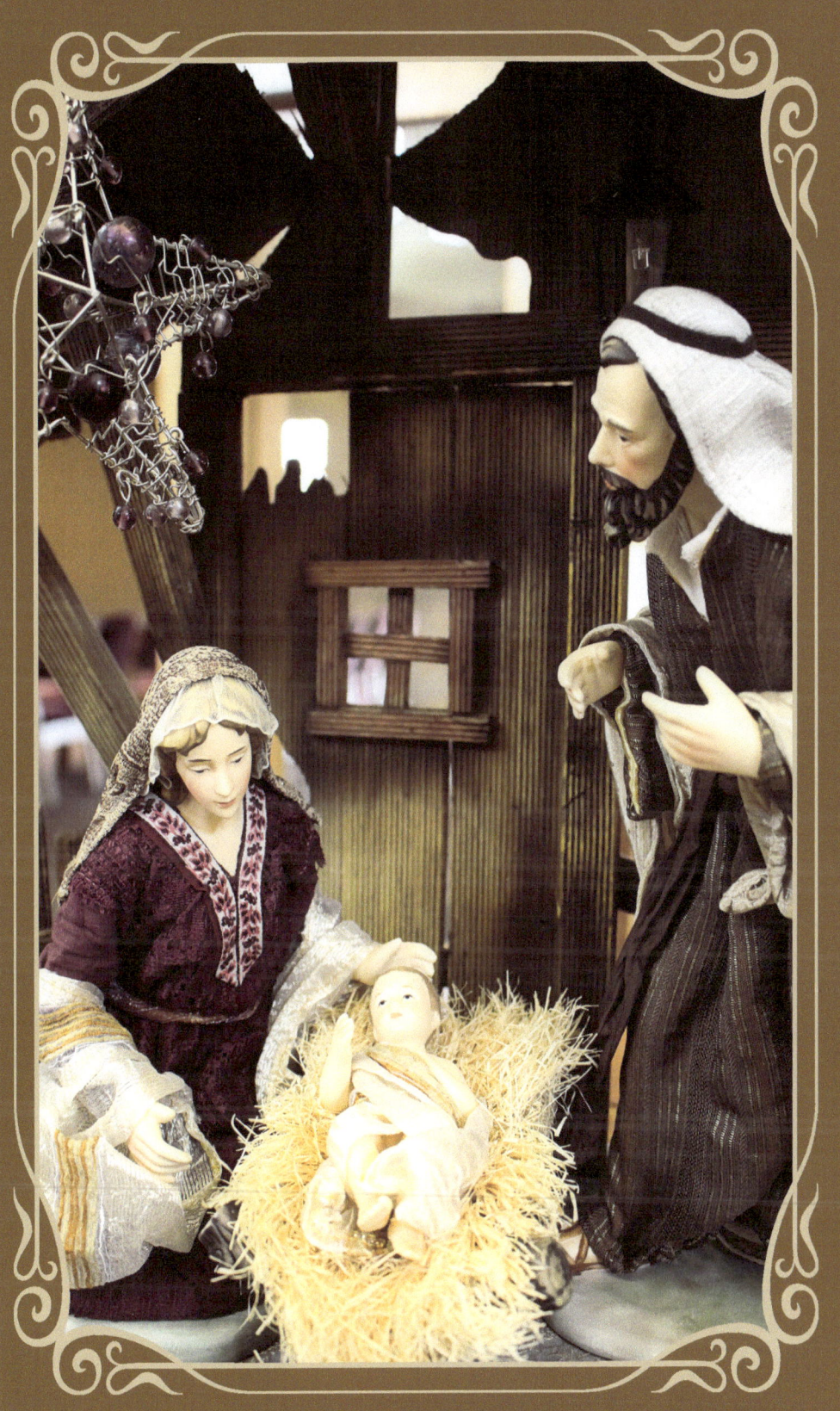

Christmas Wreath

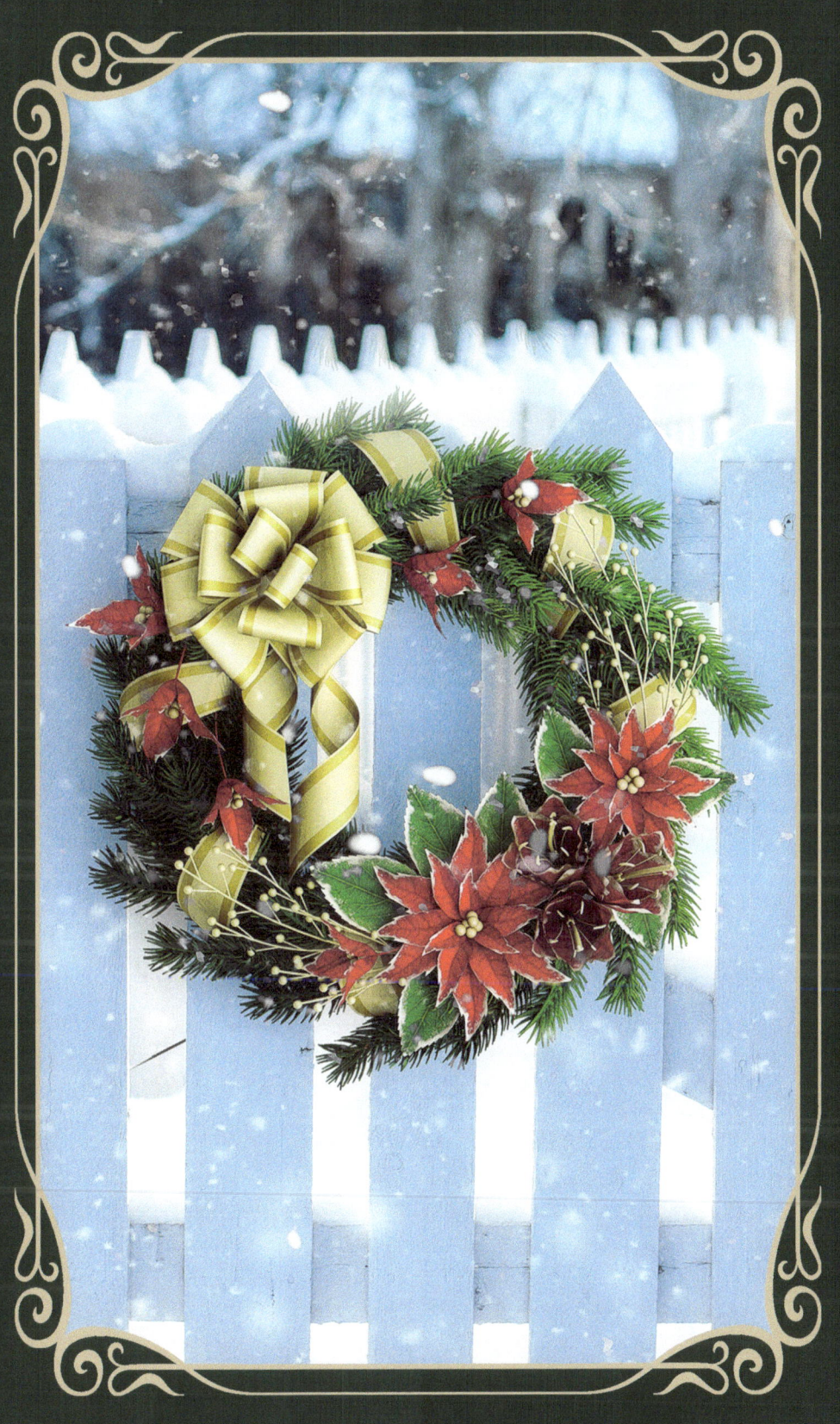